COMPREHENSIVE

THYROID DIET WITH A MEAL PLAN

FOR BEGINNERS

A simple weight-loss guide with a meal plan for hypothyroidism and Hashimoto's relief to improve your overall health

ROBERT ANDREW

ISBN:

Printed in the United States of America

Disclaimer

This publication is designed to provide competent and reliable information regarding the subject covered. However, the views expressed in this publication are those of the author alone, and should not be taken as expert instruction or professional advice. The reader is responsible for his or her actions. The author hereby disclaims any responsibility or liability whatsoever that is incurred from the use or application of the contents of this publication by the purchaser of the reader. The purchaser or reader is hereby responsible for his or her actions.

Table of Contents

INTRODUCTION

Hypothyroidism is a disorder in which the body fails to create enough thyroid hormones, which are essential for development, metabolism, and repair. As a result, persons with an underactive thyroid may find it difficult to lose weight, adding to the difficulty.

In rare circumstances, unresolved thyroid disorders might be the source of poor fat reduction and weight control.

As a result, the first step that is frequently recommended during any weight reduction journey is for patients to repair their thyroid condition.

If you've been struggling to lose stubborn weight due to your thyroid, we'll show you some of the greatest meals and simple strategies to get your metabolism running properly and lose weight for good.

The thyroid gland is a tiny, butterfly-shaped gland in your neck. It produces and stores thyroid hormones, which have an impact on practically every cell in your body. Thyroid hormones are released into the circulation when the thyroid gland receives a signal called thyroid-stimulating hormone (TSH). When thyroid hormone levels are low, this signal is given by the pituitary gland, a tiny organ located near the base of your brain.

Even when it is sufficient for TSH, the thyroid gland does not always produce thyroid hormones. Primary hypothyroidism is the most prevalent kind of hypothyroidism.

Approximately 90% of cases of primary hypothyroidism are caused by Hashimoto's thyroiditis, an autoimmune illness in which your immune system destroys your thyroid gland by mistake.

Iodine deficiency, a hereditary disease, using certain drugs, and surgery to remove part of the thyroid are all possible causes of primary hypothyroidism.

Sometimes the thyroid gland may not get enough TSH. Secondary hypothyroidism occurs when the pituitary gland does not function adequately. Thyroid hormones are crucial. They aid in the regulation of development, cell repair, and metabolism – the process through which your body transforms food into energy. Your metabolism influences your body temperature and the pace at which you burn calories. As a result, persons with hypothyroidism frequently feel chilly and exhausted, and they may gain weight quickly.

DO THYROID PATIENTS GAIN WEIGHT EASILY?

The metabolism of patients who have an underactive thyroid is hampered. Our metabolic system has a significant influence on both healthy bodily functioning and the way we burn calories. As a result, if you have metabolic issues or a sluggish metabolic rate, you may acquire weight more easily and find it more difficult to lose excess kilos.

A sluggish metabolism can also bring extra health hazards, such as elevated blood pressure and cholesterol. Thus, for a healthy life, it is important to balance food and address thyroid issues. Diagnosis is also critical. The longer you wait to be diagnosed, the more weight you are likely to acquire.

HOW DOES HYPOTHYROIDISM AFFECT YOUR METABOLISM?

The thyroid hormone regulates the rate of your metabolism. The more calories your body burns at rest, the quicker your metabolism. Hypothyroid people produce less thyroid hormone. They have a slower metabolism and burn fewer calories at rest.

A sluggish metabolism poses several health hazards. It may make you sleepy, raise your blood cholesterol levels, and make losing weight more difficult. If you have hypothyroidism and find it difficult to maintain your weight, consider practicing moderate or high-intensity exercise. Fast-paced walking, running, hiking, and rowing is examples of such activities.

According to research, moderate to high-intensity aerobic exercise may help improve thyroid hormone levels. As a result, your metabolism may speed up.

People suffering from hypothyroidism may benefit from boosting their protein intake as well. According to research, higher protein diets assist to speed up your metabolism.

WHICH NUTRIENTS ARE ESSENTIAL?

Several nutrients are essential for thyroid health.

Iodine

Iodine is a mineral that is required for the production of thyroid hormones. As a result, persons who are deficient in iodine may be at risk of hypothyroidism. Iodine deficiency is extremely widespread, affecting almost one-third of the global population. It is less frequent in wealthy nations like the United States, where iodized salt and iodine-rich seafood are commonly accessible.

If you are deficient in iodine, try adding iodized table salt to your meals or eating extra iodine-rich foods such as seaweed, seafood, dairy, and eggs. Iodine pills are unneeded since your food contains sufficient iodine. Some research has also suggested that consuming too much of this mineral may harm the thyroid gland.

Selenium

Selenium aids in the "activation" of thyroid hormones, allowing them to be utilized by the body. This vital mineral also has antioxidant properties, which means it may protect the thyroid gland from free radical damage.

Including selenium-rich foods in your diet is an excellent method to increase your selenium levels. Brazil nuts, tuna, sardines, eggs, and legumes are examples. However, unless suggested by a healthcare expert, avoid taking a selenium supplement. Supplements include high dosages of selenium, which can be dangerous in big quantities.

Zinc

Zinc, like selenium, assists the body in "activating" thyroid hormones.

Zinc may also assist the body to regulate TSH, the hormone that informs the thyroid gland when to produce thyroid hormones, according to research. Zinc deficiency is uncommon in modern nations since zinc is abundant in the diet.

If you have hypothyroidism, you should consume more zinc-rich foods such as oysters and other shellfish, beef, and chicken.

WHY IS DIET SO IMPORTANT WITH HYPOTHYROIDISM?

Nutrition is always essential to one's overall health. It is especially crucial for thyroid disease patients since poor nutrition can lead to poor thyroid function in the first place.

Your metabolism is less efficient if you have hypothyroidism. This is because your thyroid hormones (T3 and T4) control when your cells know to convert food into energy. Because hypothyroidism lowers your metabolism, you will experience unexplained weight gain.

Many people want to lose weight while dealing with an underactive thyroid. A hypothyroidism diet is crucial for more reasons than just losing weight.

90% of hypothyroidism cases are caused by Hashimoto's disease, an autoimmune illness caused by:

- Hormone disproportion

- Lack of nutrients (especially iodine)
- Food intolerance
- Leaky intestine syndrome
- Tick-borne illnesses and other long-term infections
- Exposure to toxins

When paired with a specific therapy strategy with your functional healthcare physician, treating the underlying causes of Hashimoto's can permanently correct your hypothyroidism. Your diet is one of the most essential improvements you can make to reverse your hypothyroidism. When paired with a specific therapy strategy with your functional healthcare physician, treating the underlying causes of Hashimoto's can permanently correct your hypothyroidism. Your diet is one of the most essential improvements you can make to reverse your hypothyroidism.

AIP DIET FOR HYPOTHYROIDISM

The Autoimmune Paleo (AIP) Diet is the hypothyroidism diet we recommend to our patients. Similar to the Whole30 diet, the AIP diet restricts your intake of potential food allergens.

THIS THYROID DIET IS SHORT-TERM. WHY?

This is an extremely limited diet, intending to identify any probable food sensitivities through elimination. If your hypothyroidism symptoms improve while on the AIP diet, we recommend gradually reintroducing one meal at a time. If a reintroduced meal worsens your symptoms, eliminate that food allergy from your diet completely.

WHICH NUTRIENTS ARE DANGEROUS?

Several nutrients may be harmful to hypothyroid patients' health.

Goitrogens

Goitrogens are substances that can disrupt the thyroid gland's natural function.

They acquire their name from the term goiter, which refers to an enlarged thyroid gland caused by hypothyroidism.

Surprisingly, goitrogens are found in many popular meals, including:

• Soy foods, such as tofu, tempeh, and edamame

• Certain vegetables, such as cabbage, broccoli, kale, cauliflower, spinach, and so on.

• Fruits and starchy plants, such as sweet potatoes, cassava, peaches, and strawberries.

• Nuts and seeds, such as millet, pine nuts, and peanuts

In theory, hypothyroid patients should avoid goitrogens. However, this appears to be a concern mainly for persons who are deficient in iodine or consume a lot of goitrogens.

Cooking meals containing goitrogens may also inactivate these chemicals.

Pearl millet is an exception to the list above. According to certain research, pearl millet may interfere with thyroid function even if you do not have an iodine shortage.

FOODS TO AVOID IF YOU SUFFER FROM HYPOTHYROIDISM

If you have hypothyroidism, you don't have to avoid many foods. Goitrogen-containing meals, on the other hand, should be consumed in moderation and, ideally, prepared.

You should avoid consuming highly processed meals because they are often rich in calories. If you have hypothyroidism, this might be an issue since you may gain weight easily.

The following foods and supplements should be avoided:

- **Millet**: any kind

- **Highly processed meals**, such as hot dogs, cakes, and cookies

- **Supplements:** Adequate selenium and iodine intakes are required for thyroid health, but too much of either can be harmful. Supplement with selenium and iodine only if directed by a healthcare expert.

Here is a list of foods that may be consumed in moderation. If ingested in high quantities, the following foods contain goitrogens or are recognized irritants:

- Soy-based foods such as tofu, tempeh, edamame beans, soy milk, and so on.

- Peaches, pears, and strawberries are examples of fruits.

- Beverages: coffee, green tea, and alcohol may aggravate your thyroid gland.

FOODS TO EAT IF YOU HAVE HYPOTHYROIDISM

If you have hypothyroidism, you have several dietary alternatives, including:

- Eggs: whole eggs are preferable since the yolk has the most iodine and selenium, while the whites are high in protein.

- Meat: any meat, including lamb, beef, and chicken.

- Fish: any type of fish, including salmon, tuna, halibut, shrimp, and so on.

- Vegetables: all vegetables — cruciferous vegetables in moderation, especially when cooked

- Fruits: all other fruits, such as berries, bananas, oranges, tomatoes, and so on.

- Grain and gluten-free seed options include rice, buckwheat, quinoa, chia seeds, and flax seeds.

- Dairy: all dairy products such as milk, cheese, yogurt, and so on.

- Drinks: water and non-caffeinated beverages

Hypothyroid patients should consume a diet high in vegetables, fruits, and lean meats. These are low in calories and filling, which may aid in weight loss.

WHAT FOODS HELP WITH HYPOTHYROIDISM?

If you experience signs of an underactive thyroid, it might be an indication of hypothyroidism, a kind of thyroid illness. You may have heard that foods like coconut oil can assist enhance thyroid hormone production if you have hypothyroidism (your thyroid gland does not create enough hormones). However, there is no medical evidence to suggest that these meals will benefit an underactive thyroid.

Instead, the best course of action is to stick to the medical treatment (such as thyroid hormone replacement) that your healthcare physician has suggested.

Is there anything I should avoid when taking hypothyroidism medication? If you're using synthetic thyroid hormones to treat an underactive thyroid, avoid taking them at the same time as the following meals and supplements, and instead space them out by a few hours:

• Soybean flour • Cottonseed meal

• Iron supplements or iron-containing multivitamins • Calcium supplements

Other prescription drugs may potentially interfere with your thyroid medication, so make sure to review all of your prescriptions with your doctor.

WHAT FOODS ARE BENEFICIAL TO HYPERTHYROIDISM?

There is no single diet that can immediately improve your hyperthyroid symptoms. However, if Graves' disease is the cause of your hyperthyroidism (the most frequent cause of an overactive thyroid), then eating particular foods will assist boost your immune system health and hence overall thyroid function. Among these foods are:

- Dairy products, orange juice, eggs, salmon, or other calcium and/or vitamin D-fortified foods, since Grave's disease can cause bone loss and osteoporosis, and these foods can help avoid these difficulties.

- Protein-rich meals, such as chicken, turkey, beans, and nuts, because weight loss is a major sign of hyperthyroidism, and these foods can help keep your present muscle mass while potentially assisting in weight gain.

Kale, Brussels sprouts, radishes, and cauliflower are examples of cruciferous vegetables. They may restrict your thyroid gland's capacity to digest iodine and generate thyroid hormones, potentially alleviating hyperthyroidism symptoms. They are also known as goitrogenic foods (foods that can help suppress thyroid hormone production). However, if you have an autoimmune disorder such as Graves' disease, you should exercise caution with these veggies and consult with your healthcare professional before including them in your diet.

WHAT FOODS ARE ADVERSE FOR THYROID FUNCTION?

Now that we've covered foods to eat to improve thyroid function, let's look at foods to avoid if you have a thyroid problem.

If you have hypothyroidism, avoid meals high in soy protein since they may interfere with your body's capacity to absorb replacement thyroid hormones.

You may have also heard that cruciferous vegetables such as spinach, kale, cabbage, cauliflower, broccoli, turnips, and Brussels sprouts should be avoided.

It's critical to understand that certain meals, on their own, are unlikely to affect your thyroid function. They are called goitrogenic foods, however, since they interfere with your thyroid's capacity to absorb iodine, which can reduce thyroid hormone production and raise your risk of goiter.

What does this imply for you? If you aren't receiving enough iodine in your diet, or if you know you have low iodine levels, talk to your doctor about avoiding these veggies.

However, if you have hypothyroidism or a family history of goiters (an enlarged thyroid gland), you don't have to avoid these veggies. Instead, attempt to vary your vegetable servings throughout the day so that you don't consume too many goitrogens in a single meal. Also, juicing these veggies greatly increases their content of thiocyanates, the chemical in goitrogenic vegetables that interferes with thyroid gland function.

If you're currently taking synthetic thyroid hormones for thyroid dysfunction, you generally don't need to worry about eating cruciferous veggies (though it's a good idea to discuss it with your doctor). Instead, concentrate on eating a well-balanced diet that is high in the vitamins and nutrients you require. This will assist you in keeping your entire body, not just your thyroid, in good operating order.

WHAT FOODS SHOULD YOU AVOID IF YOU HAVE HYPERTHYROIDISM?

If you have hyperthyroidism, reducing your intake of specific foods, such as:

- Caffeine, which may aggravate hyperthyroidism symptoms including agitation, anxiety, and weight loss.

- Common food allergens, including corn and gluten, since these may trigger worsening symptoms. So consider talking with your healthcare provider about a gluten-free diet—or other specialized diets—if you have hyperthyroidism.

HOW DOES THYROID DISEASE OCCUR?

Iodine is required by the thyroid to produce hormones, although the two have a troubled relationship. So, because the blood cannot contain that much iodine, the thyroid must look for and absorb every trace of it in the blood.

Iodine is a hazardous element that is seldom found in nature. When iodine is found in food, water, cosmetics, and practically every other source, it is in its less reactive form, iodide. The thyroid gland subsequently converts the iodide into the more volatile iodine to produce thyroid hormones. The thyroid reacts to it in the same way that a scientist would react to a strong acid, coating its cells with antioxidants such as glutathione for protection. If iodine leaks, the thyroid cells become irritated and unable to produce hormones efficiently. The immune system might then target the inflamed cells, killing them and exacerbating a person's thyroid hormone deficiency. Regardless, it all starts with too much iodine.

We used to believe that thyroid illness was incurable. We now know that until virtually all of the cells are dead, the harm may be prevented and the cells healed if the cells are not exposed to excessive iodine. We cannot and should not reduce our iodine intake to zero. Iodine is found in almost every diet. However, research experiments show that even a little reduction in iodine consumption is typically enough to treat thyroid illness.

The Thyroid Reset Diet reduces a person's iodine intake sufficiently to allow the thyroid to clean out the excess iodine that has slowed it down; the diet accomplishes this by eliminating hidden sources of iodine in your meals.

HOW CAN I NATURALLY CURE MY THYROID CONDITION?

If a thyroid test and physician examination reveal that you have a thyroid issue, you must follow the medical recommendations of your healthcare practitioner. It is not feasible to repair your thyroid just by changing your diet.

However, this does not exclude you from making lifestyle adjustments that will naturally improve your thyroid health and help you manage a thyroid malfunction. First and foremost, concentrate on eating a nutritious diet, since this will continue to provide advantages even after your thyroid hormone levels have been regulated owing to medical therapy.

Also, because both hypothyroidism and hyperthyroidism alter the way your body metabolizes food, increasing your fiber intake can help with digestion. Whole grains, fruits, and vegetables are examples of fiber-rich foods. Make sure you're getting enough nutrients, and choose proteins from lean sources like fish or plant-based choices like beans or nuts. You should also consume healthy fats such as olive oil and omega-3 fatty acids.

Naturally regulating your thyroid health also entails avoiding harmful meals. Avoid "bad fats" such as trans fats, which are commonly present in goods such as margarine, processed meals, and hydrogenated oils.

IMPORTANT NUTRIENTS FOR HEALTHY THYROID FUNCTION

There are several vital nutrients that hypothyroidism patients should make sure to get into their diets:

- Iodine, which is contained in iodized table salt, is required for thyroid hormone synthesis. The most prevalent cause of goiters – an enlarged thyroid — is iodine insufficiency. Iodine appears to be useful in the treatment and prevention of autoimmune illnesses like Hashimoto's thyroiditis.

- Selenium is present naturally in muscle meats, seafood, Brazil nuts, and eggs, as well as in supplements.

According to research, adding selenium to a traditional hypothyroidism medication enhances thyroid function.

- Vitamin D is required for thyroid function. A lack of vitamin D can result in Hashimoto's disease and hypothyroidism. Fish, cow liver, and egg yolks are all high in vitamin D. Sunlight exposure is our best source of Vitamin D. Please visit our online store for high-quality, third-party-tested Vitamin D.
- Zinc aids in the conversion of T4 to T3, which is vital in the prevention of thyroid diseases. Higher T3 levels are associated with adequate zinc consumption. Dietary zinc may be obtained through meats, shellfish, and

mollusks. Check out our Prime Zinc for medical quality, third-party verified zinc.

- Probiotics are beneficial microorganisms that may be found in sauerkraut, kombucha, and supplements. Probiotics have been shown in studies to help reverse leaky gut by strengthening the lining of your intestines. If you have the leaky gut syndrome, dietary probiotics can help you regain normal thyroid function.

SUPPLEMENT & MEDICATION CONSIDERATIONS

Depending on your Hashimoto's triggers, some dietary supplements may help reduce hypothyroidism symptoms:

- **Iodine supplements** — if you are at risk of iodine deficiency
- **Selenium**
- **Zinc** – click here for a medical grade, 3rd party tested Zinc
- **Vitamin D3** — especially if your kidneys are underactive, or you don't go outside much
- **Vitamin B complex**
- **Probiotics** — if you are at risk of leaky gut
- **Curcumin** — since it helps prevent autoimmune diseases, such as Hashimoto's
- **Chasteberry** — because it balances hormones
- **Ashwagandha**

However, there are several foods, supplements, and medications that you should avoid while on thyroid medication (such as thyroid hormone replacement).

If you are taking thyroid medication (such as levothyroxine), avoid these foods/drugs within several hours of your thyroid medication and see your doctor:

- Walnuts
- Soybean meal
- Cottonseed oil
- Fiber excess (can impede digestion of important nutrients)
- Excess iodine (may cause Graves' disease and, as a result, hyperthyroidism in some persons)
- Calcium supplementation

- Iron supplementation
- Some ulcer treatments, such as sucralfate
- Cholesterol-lowering medications such as cholestyramine or colestipol
- Calcium, magnesium, or aluminum-containing antacids

CAN YOUR DIET HELP REGULATE HYPOTHYROIDISM?

While a high-quality diet can assist balance hormone activity and improve thyroid management, it should be highlighted that food alone cannot treat hypothyroidism. However, eating the correct meals that provide adequate nutrition, exercise, and any medicine that you may have been prescribed will help reduce your symptoms.

Weight reduction will be simpler if your thyroid is steady and you have more control over your lifestyle. A proper thyroid-controlling diet also takes into account your body's capacity to burn calories, and nutrients, metabolize and avoid dietary sensitivities. However, it is critical to include nutrient-rich meals such as:

Increase your iodine intake According to statistics, one-third of the world's population is deficient in iodine. Iodine is another vital element that aids in the stimulation of thyroid function in the body. As a result, if you have hypothyroidism, be sure to supplement your diet with iodine, which will stimulate TSH production in the body. Foods such as table salt, seafood, dairy, and eggs can be quite beneficial.

It is important to consume fiber.

One of the greatest methods for thyroid sufferers to reduce weight is to consume enough fiber. Fiber aids in the regulation of digestion, the removal of harmful pollutants, and, most critically, the control of calorie intake. Make sure to include lots of fruits, vegetables, and legumes in your regular diet. Supplements may be explored as well.

Consume more selenium-rich foods.

Selenium is another crucial trace element that aids the body in producing an abundance of TSH hormones. A sufficient amount of selenium in your diet can also aid in the elimination of free radicals, which lead to weight gain. Certain studies have also shown that selenium can improve immunological function in the body.

Consider including selenium-rich foods such as Brazil nuts, sardines, eggs, and various types of legumes in your diet.

Limit your Consumption of sugar and high-carb foods

Sugar and high-carbohydrate diets are enemies of weight loss. As a result, if you wish to regulate your thyroid and lose weight effectively, try restricting or eliminating sugar sources from your diet. High-starchy carbohydrate meals, which might add sugar, are bad for you. Consider including foods with a low glycemic index that do not boost insulin levels. Many people are now considering the Paleo diet, which entails eating a low-sugar, whole-food diet.

Likewise, some people benefit from a low-carbohydrate diet, such as the

Ketogenic diet.

Eat more anti-inflammatory foods

Foods that assist the body to reduce active inflammation or autoimmune processes that might impair thyroid function can also help thyroid patients lose weight faster. An anti-inflammatory diet may also be beneficial.

Include more gluten-free products

Many studies have found a relationship between gluten sensitivity and autoimmune disorders including Hashimoto's thyroiditis, which can result in an underactive thyroid. As a result, switching to gluten-free food may help some people manage their hypothyroidism and lose weight.

Consider changing the timing of your meals

Changing the time of your meals is one of the simplest methods to speed up your metabolism and burn fat faster. Many thyroid patients benefit by fasting, limiting the number of meals they eat per day or eating them at specific times. Fasting can also help reduce cravings, and processed food intake, and control hunger hormones. Remember to address any flaws ahead of time.

Hydrate well

Hydration is essential for weight reduction and is one of the simplest ways to keep hormones in balance. Adequate water consumption will help reduce water retention, enhance digestion, and aid in the evacuation of toxins from the body. It may also suppress your appetite. If you've hit a weight loss plateau or are having difficulty losing weight, drinking more water may help.

ARE THERE EXERCISES THAT CAN HELP?

Exercise is an important part of having a healthy lifestyle. Several studies have now demonstrated that specific activities can assist regulate thyroid function in the body while also enhancing metabolic function. If you have hypothyroidism and want to reduce weight, you should exercise for at least one hour every day.

Prioritizing the type of exercise you undertake might also be beneficial. Strength training, muscle-building activities, lifting weights, and Pilates, for example, maybe more

	Breakfast	Lunch	Dinner
Monday		Cannellini Bean Salad	Quick Moussaka
Tuesday	Tomato and Watermelon Salad	Edgy Veggie Wraps	Spicy Tomato Baked Eggs
Wednesday	Blueberry Oats Bowl	Carrot, Orange, and Avocado Salad	Salmon with Potatoes and Corn Salad
Thursday	Banana Yogurt Pots	Mixed Bean Salad	Spiced Carrot and Lentil Soup
Friday	Tomato and Watermelon Salad	Panzanella Salad	Med Chicken, Quinoa, and Greek Salad
Saturday	Blueberry Oats Bowl	Quinoa and Stir Fried Veg	Grilled Vegetables with Bean Mash

Sunday	Banana Yogurt Pots	Moroccan Chickpea Soup	Spicy Mediterranean Beet Salad

beneficial than basic cardio in managing TSH levels and maximizing weight reduction.

7DAYS HYPERTHYROIDISM DIET MEAL PLAN

In the meal plan are recipes for breakfast, lunch, and dinner.

Snacks are recommended between meal times. Some good snacks include:

- A handful of nuts or seeds
- A piece of fruit
- Carrots or baby carrots
- Berries or grapes

Day 1: Monday

Breakfast: Banana Yogurt Pots

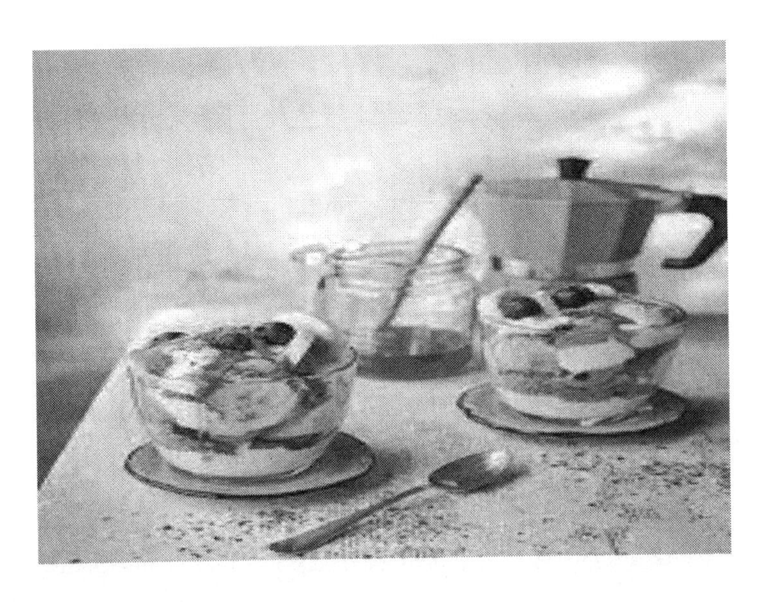

Nutrition

- 236 Calories
- 14g Protein
- 32g Carbs
- Fat - 7g

Prep time: 5 minutes

Ingredients (for 2 people)

- 225g Greek yogurt
- 2 bananas, sliced into chunks
- 15g walnuts, toasted and chopped

Instructions

1. Place some of the yogurts into the bottom of a glass. Add a layer of banana, then yogurt, and repeat. Once the glass is full, scatter with the nuts.

Lunch: Cannellini Bean Salad

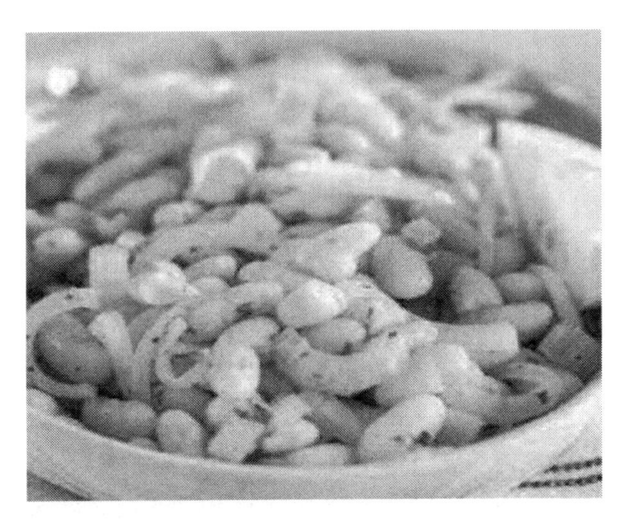

Nutrition

- Calories – 302
- Protein – 20g
- Carbohydrates – 54g
- Fat – 0g

Prep time: 5 minutes

Ingredients (for 2 people)

- 600g canned cannellini beans
- 70g cherry tomatoes, halved
- ½ red onion, thinly sliced
- ½ tablespoon red wine vinegar
- small bunch of basil, torn

Instructions

1. Rinse and drain the beans and mix with the tomatoes, onion, and vinegar. Season, then add basil just before serving.

Dinner: Quick'n'Easy Moussaka

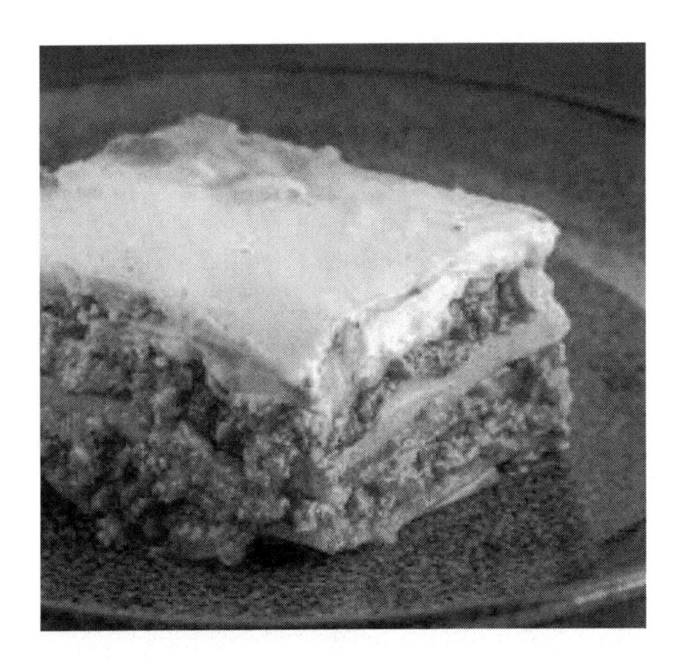

Nutrition

- 577 Calories
- 27g Protein
- Carbs – 46g
- Fat – 27g

Prep time + cook time: 30 minutes

Ingredients (for 2 people)

- 1 tablespoon extra virgin olive oil
- ½ onion, finely chopped
- 1 garlic clove, finely chopped
- 250g lean beef mince
- 200g can of chopped tomatoes
- 1 tablespoon tomato purée
- 1 teaspoon ground cinnamon
- 200 g canned chickpeas
- 100g crumbled feta cheese pack
- Mint (fresh preferable)
- To serve, brown bread

Instructions

1. Heat the oil in a skillet. Fry the onion and garlic until tender. Fry the mince for 3-4 minutes, or until browned.

2. Add the tomatoes to the pan, along with the tomato purée and cinnamon, and season with salt and pepper. Allow the mince to cook for 20 minutes. Halfway through, add the chickpeas.

2. Top the mince with the feta and mint. With toasted bread, serve.

Day 2: Tuesday

Breakfast: Tomato and Watermelon Salad

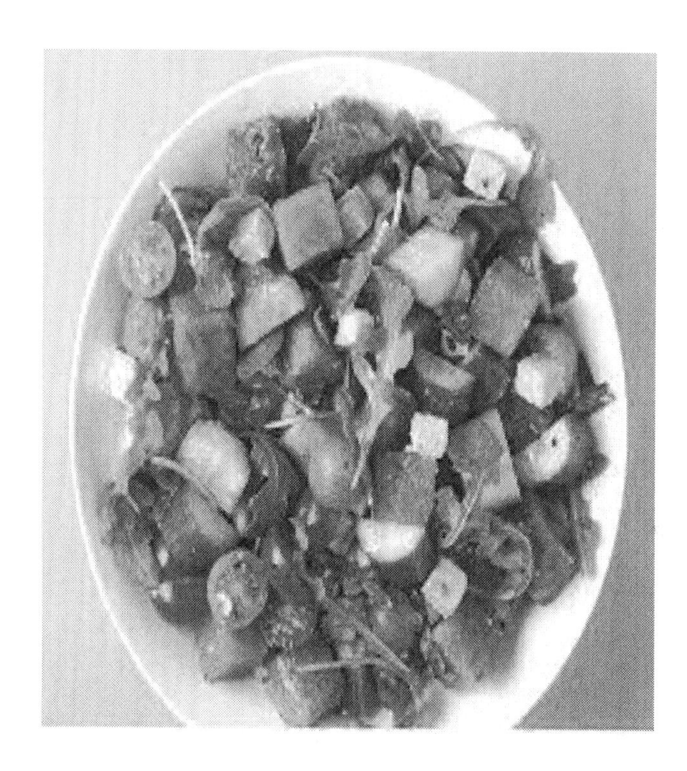

Nutrition

- 177 calories
- 5g protein
- 3g Carbohydrates
- Fat - 13g

Prep time + cook time: 5 minutes

Ingredients (for 2 people)

- 1 tablespoon olive oil
- 1 tablespoon red wine vinegar
- 14 teaspoon chili flakes
- 1 tablespoon chopped mint
- 120g chopped tomatoes

- 250g watermelon, diced
- 50g crumbled feta cheese

Instructions

1. To make the dressing, whisk together the oil, vinegar, chili flakes, and mint, then season.

3. Combine the tomatoes and melons in a mixing basin. Pour over the dressing, top with the feta, and serve.

Lunch: Edgy Veggie Wraps

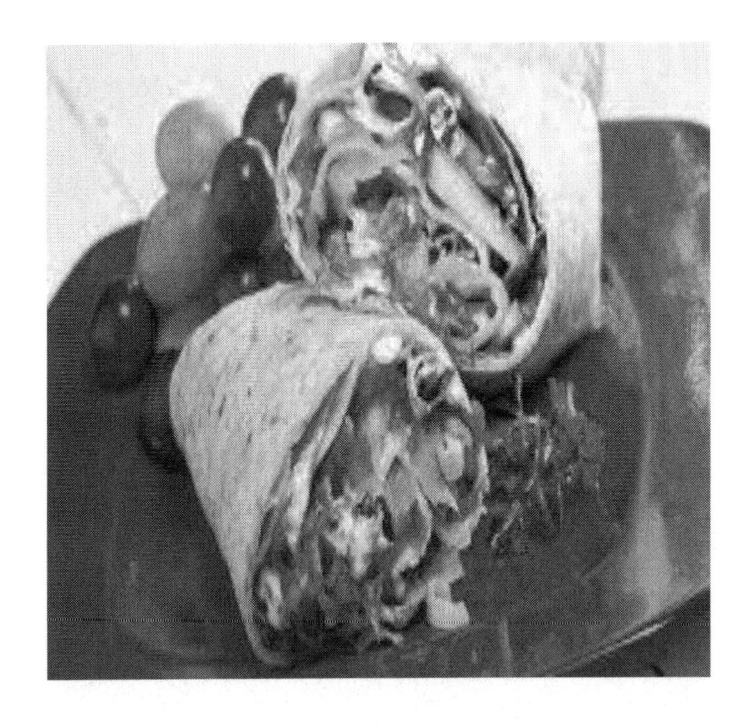

Nutrition

- 310 calories
- 11g protein
- Carbohydrates - 39g
- Fat - 11g

Prep time + cook time: 10 minutes

Ingredients (for 2 people)

- 100 grams of cherry tomatoes
- One cucumber
- 6 olives, Kalamata
- 2 wholemeal tortilla wraps
- 50 grams feta cheese

- 2 tablespoons houmous

Instructions

1. Chop the tomatoes, slice the cucumber into sticks, divide the olives, and remove the stones from the olives.

2. Warm the tortillas.

4. Spread the houmous on top of the wrap. Place the veggie mixture in the center and roll up.

Dinner: Spicy Tomato Baked Eggs

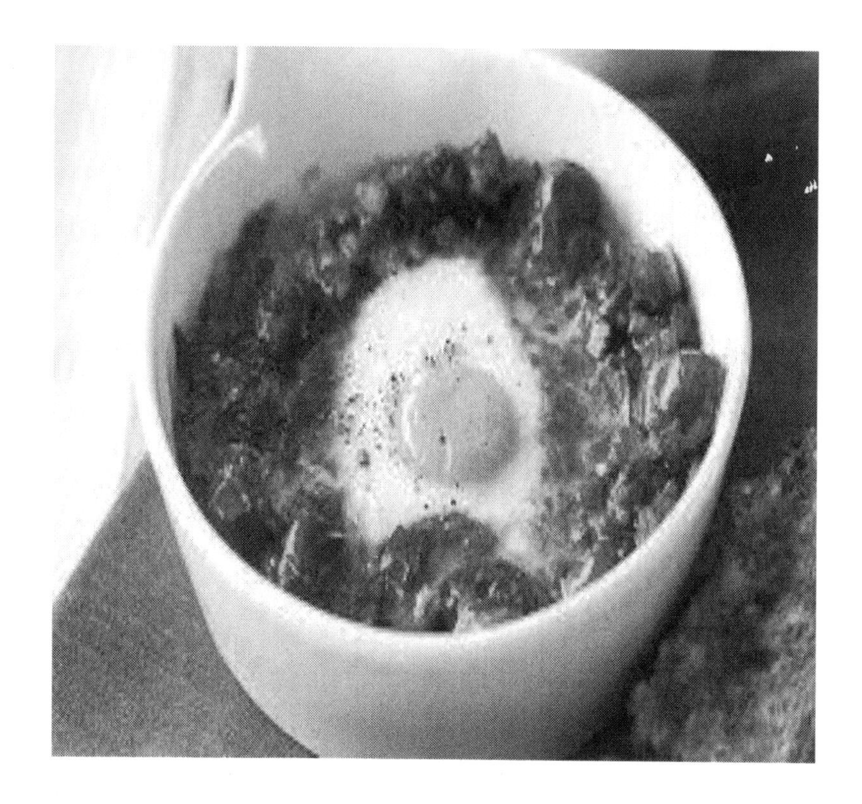

Nutrition

- 417 calories
- 19g protein
- Carbohydrates - 45g
- Fat - 17g

Prep time + cook time: 25 minutes

Ingredients (for 2 people)

- 1 tablespoon olive oil
- 2 chopped red onions
- 1 deseeded and chopped red chili
- 1 chopped garlic clove
- coriander, small bunch, stems and leaves chopped separately
- 800g tinned cherry tomatoes
- 4 eggs
- brown bread for serving

Instructions

1. In a frying pan with a cover, heat the oil and sauté the onions, chili, garlic, and coriander stems for 5 minutes, or until tender. Stir in the tomatoes and cook for 8-10 minutes.

2. Make four dips in the sauce using the back of a big spoon, then crack an egg into each one. Cover the pan and simmer for 6-8 minutes, or until the eggs are done to your preference. Serve with toast and garnished with coriander leaves.

Day 3: Wednesday

Breakfast: Blueberry Oats Bowl

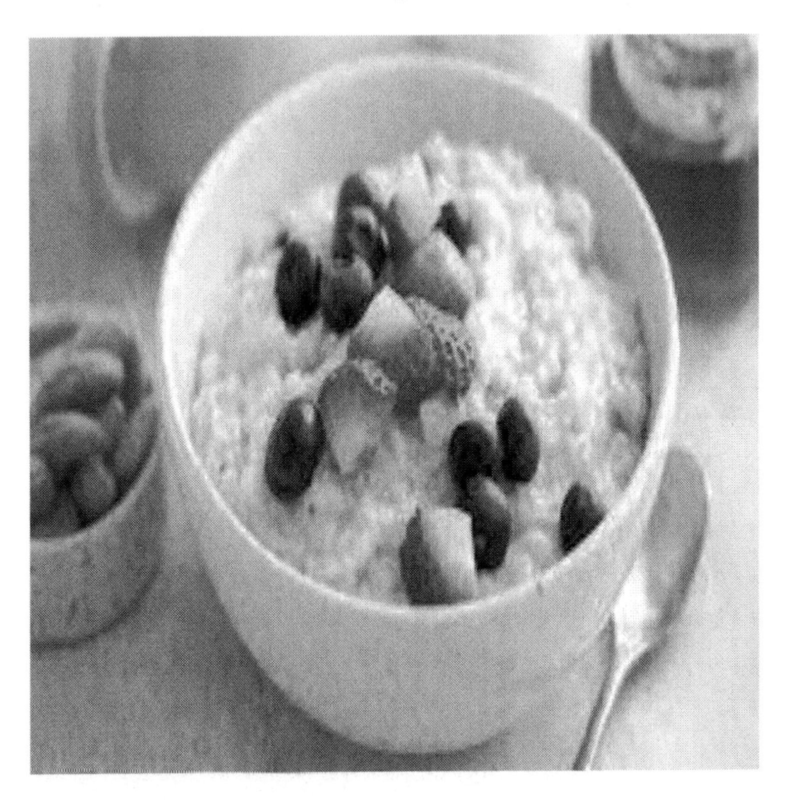

Nutrition

- 235 calories
- 13g protein
- Carbohydrates - 38g
- Fat - 4g

Prep time + cook time: 10 minutes

Ingredients (for 2 people)

- 60g oat porridge
- Greek yogurt (160g)
- 175 grams of blueberries
- 1 teaspoon honey

Instructions

1. Combine the oats and 400ml of water in a saucepan. For about 2 minutes, heat and stir. Remove

from heat and stir in a third of the yogurt.

2. Combine the blueberries, honey, and 1 tbsp of water in a saucepan. Poach the blueberries gently until they are soft.

3. Divide the porridge among the dishes and top with the remaining yogurt and blueberries.

Lunch: Carrot, Orange and Avocado Salad

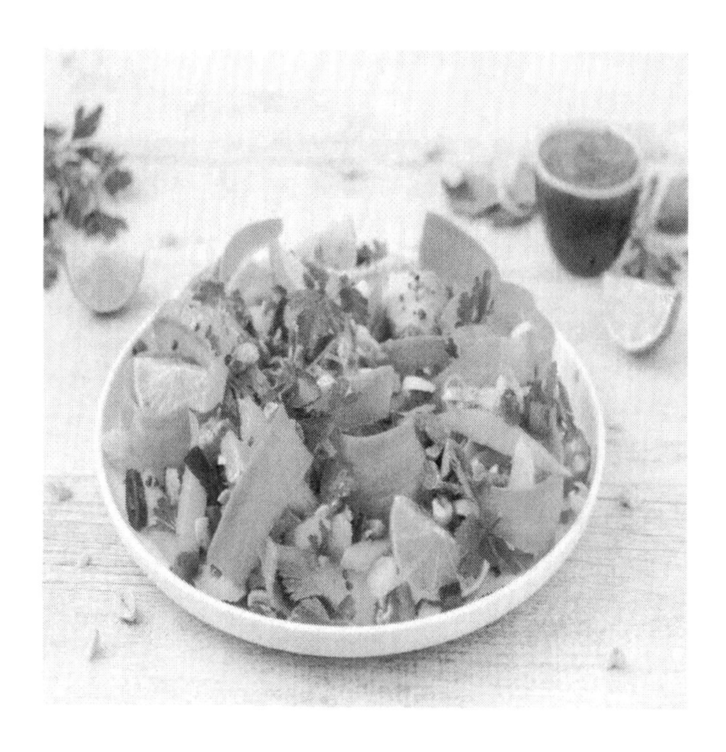

Nutrition

177 calories

- 5g protein
- 13g Carbohydrates
- Fat - 13g

Prep time + cook time: 5 minutes

Ingredients (for 2 people)

- 1 orange, plus 1 orange's zest and juice
- 2 carrots, cut in half lengthwise and sliced with a peeler
- 35g rocket/arugula pack
- 1 stoned, peeled, and sliced avocado

- 1 tablespoon olive oil

Instructions

Combine the orange segments, carrots, rocket, and avocado in a mixing dish. Combine the orange juice, zest, and oil in a mixing bowl. Season the salad with salt and pepper.

Dinner: Salmon with Potatoes and Corn Salad

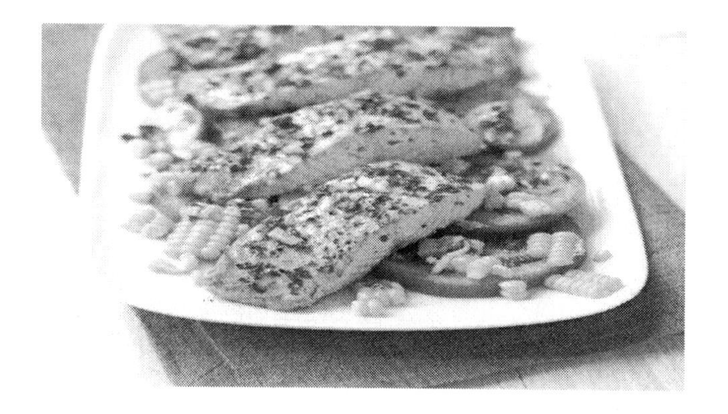

Nutrition

- 479 calories
- 43g protein
- Carbohydrates - 27g
- Fat - 21g

Prep time + cook time: 30 minutes

Ingredients (for 2 people)

- 200g young baby potatoes
- 1 ear of sweetcorn
- 2 fillets of skinless salmon
- 60g tomato
- 1 tablespoon red wine vinegar

1 tablespoon extra-virgin olive oil

- 1 finely chopped shallot
- 1 tbsp coarsely chopped capers
- a few basil leaves

Instructions

1. Boil potatoes until soft, then add corn for the last 5 minutes. Drain and allow to cool.

2. To make the dressing, whisk together the vinegar, oil, shallot, capers, basil, and spice.

3. Preheat the grill to high. Rub some dressing on the fish and cook for 7-8 minutes, skin side down. Place tomatoes on a

platter. Slice the potatoes, remove the corn from the cob, and place on a platter. Drizzle the remaining dressing over the fish.

Day 4: Thursday

Breakfast: Banana Yogurt Pots

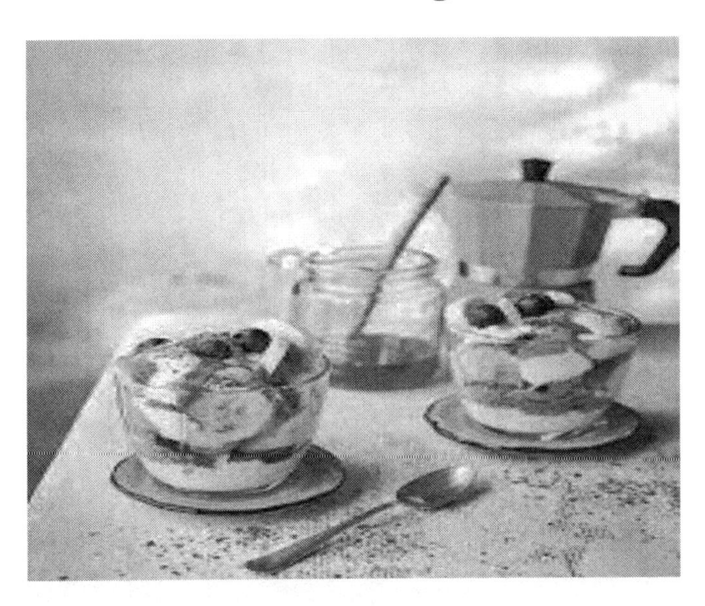

Lunch: Mixed Bean Salad

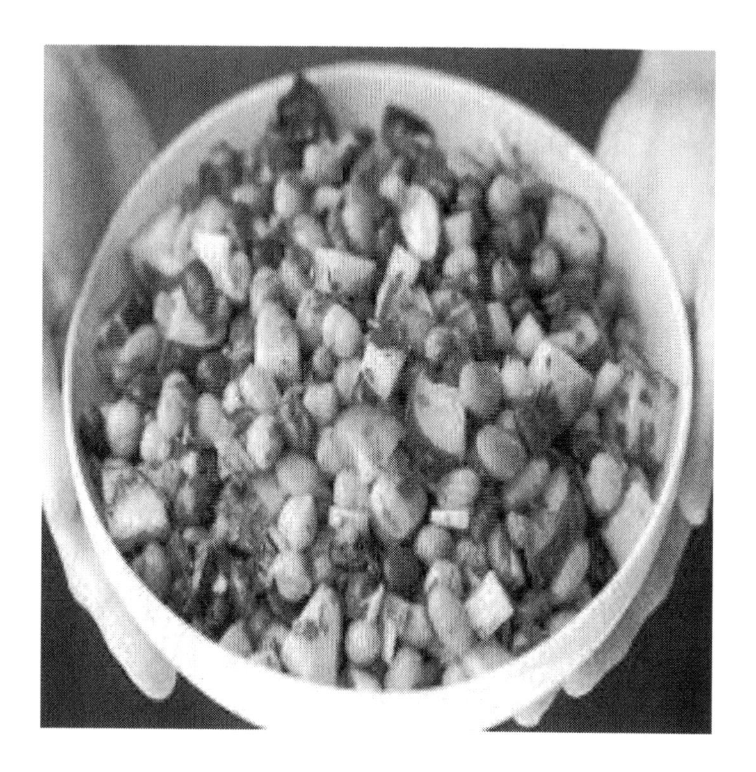

Nutrition

- 240 calories
- 11g protein

- Carbohydrates - 22g
- Fat - 12g

Prep time + cook time: 10 minutes

Ingredients (for 2 people)

- 145g artichoke heart in oil jar
- 12 tablespoons sundried tomato paste
- 12 teaspoons of red wine vinegar
- 200g cannellini beans, washed and drained
- 150g pack tomatoes, Kalamata black olives, quartered
- 2 spring onions, thinly cut diagonally

- 100g crumbled feta cheese

Instructions

1. Drain the artichokes, reserving 1-2 tablespoons of the oil. Stir in the oil, sun-dried tomato paste, and vinegar until smooth. Season with pepper to taste.

2. Chop the artichokes and place them in a basin. Combine the cannellini beans, tomatoes, olives, spring onions, and half of the feta cheese in a mixing bowl. Pour the artichoke oil mixture into a serving dish. Serve with the remaining feta cheese crumbled on top.

Dinner: Spiced Carrot and Lentil Soup

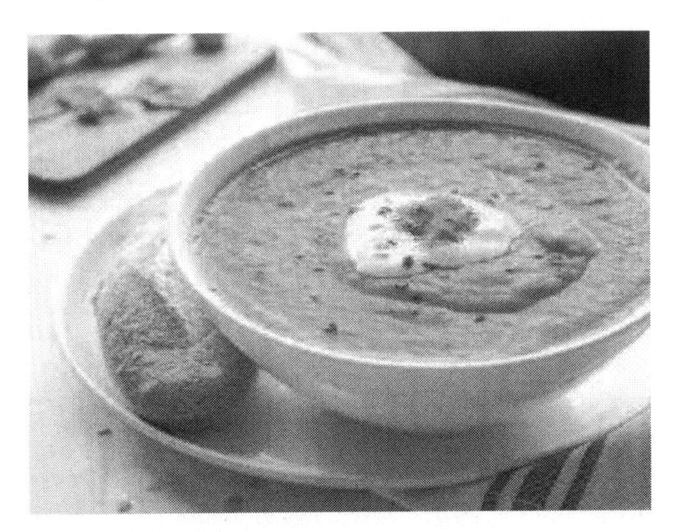

Nutrition

238 calories

- 11g protein
- Carbohydrates - 34g
- Fat - 7g

Prep time + cook time: 25 minutes

Ingredients (for 2 people)

- 1 teaspoon cumin seeds
- 1 tsp chili flakes
- 1 tablespoon olive oil
- 300g cleaned and roughly shredded carrots (no need to peel)
- 70g red split lentils
- 500ml boiling vegetable stock (from a cube is fine)
- 60ml of milk

Instructions

1. Heat a large saucepan and dry fry the cumin seeds and chili flakes for 1 minute. Scoop out about half of the seeds with a spoon and set them aside. Add the oil, carrot, lentils, stock, and milk to the pan and bring to a boil. Simmer for 15 minutes until the lentils have swollen and softened.

2. Whizz the soup with a stick blender or in a food processor until smooth. Season to taste and finish with a dollop of Greek yogurt and a sprinkling of the reserved toasted spices.

Day 5: Friday

Breakfast: Tomato and Watermelon Salad

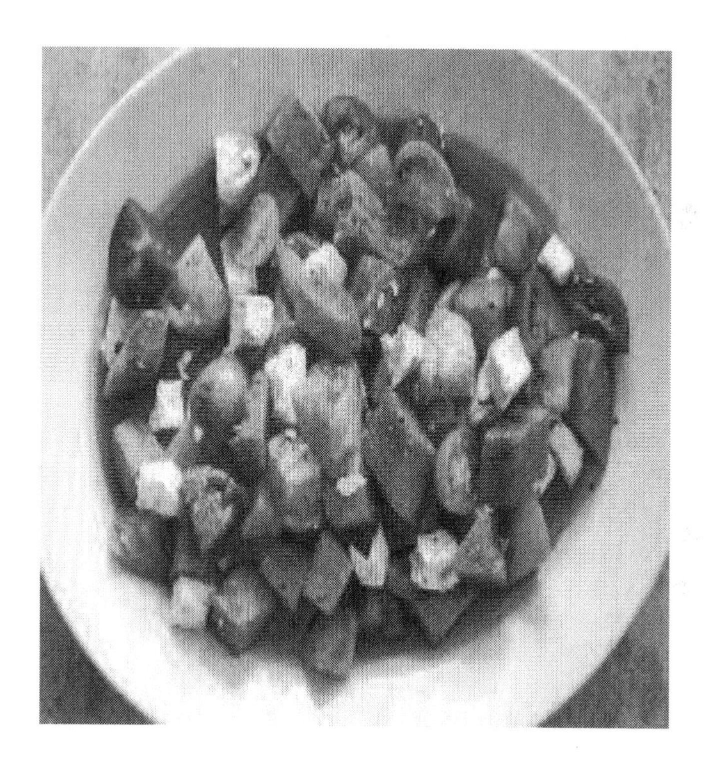

Lunch: Panzanella Salad

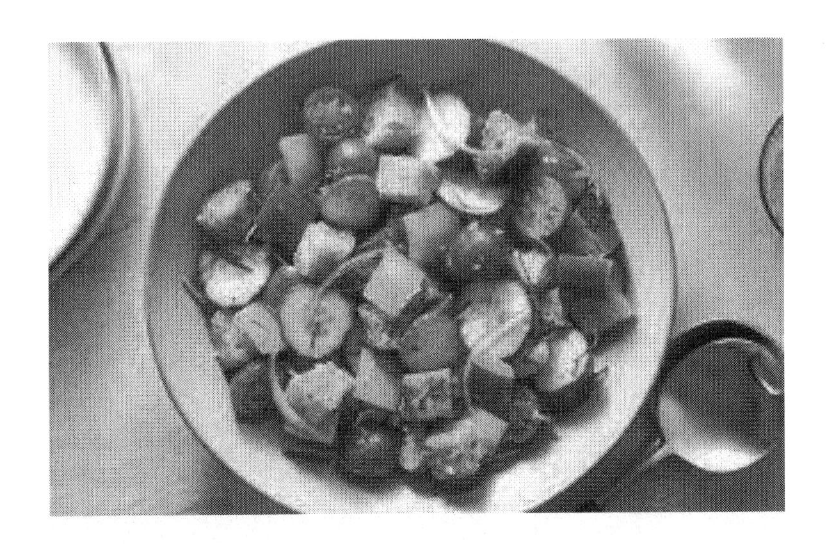

Nutrition

- 452 calories
- 6g protein
- Carbohydrates - 37g
- Fat - 25g

Prep time + cook time: 10 minutes

Ingredients (for 2 people)

- 400g tomatoes
- 1 smashed garlic clove
- 1 tablespoon capers, washed and drained
- 1 ripe avocado, peeled, stoned, and sliced
- 1 finely sliced tiny red onion
- 2 pieces of toasted bread
- 2 tablespoons olive oil
- 1 tablespoon red wine vinegar
- a few basil leaves

Instructions

1. Chop the tomatoes and place them in a mixing dish. Season to taste, then add the garlic, capers, avocado, and onion. Set aside for 10 minutes after thoroughly mixing.

2. In the meantime, tear the bread into bits and place it in a mixing basin. Drizzle half of the olive oil and half of the vinegar over the top. When ready to serve, sprinkle the tomatoes and basil leaves over the top and drizzle with the remaining oil and vinegar. Stir well before serving.

Dinner: Med Chicken, Quinoa, and Greek Salad

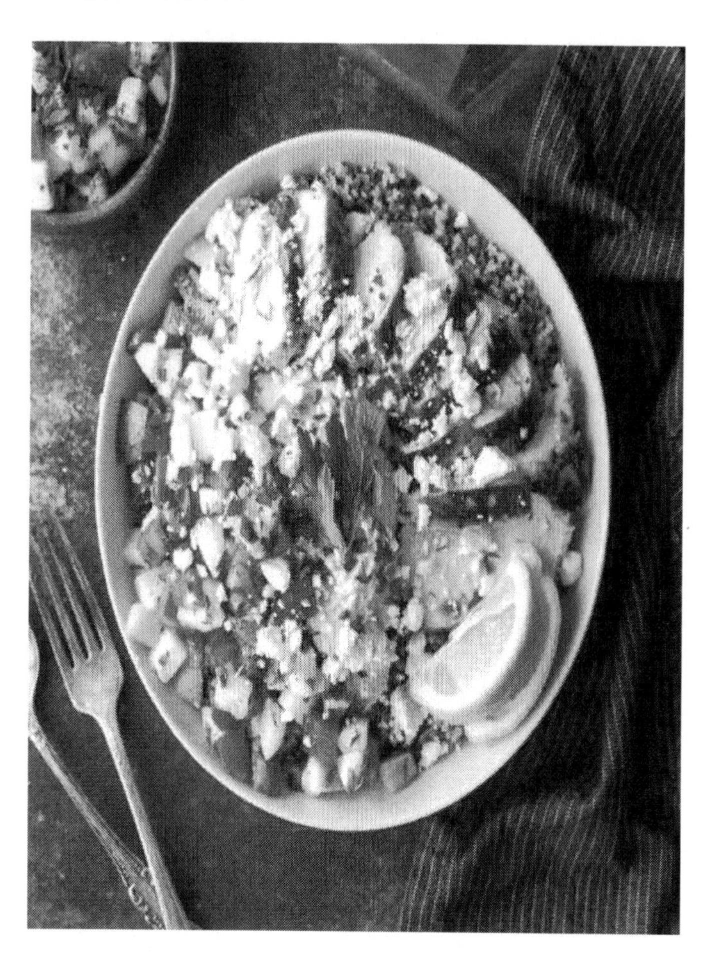

Nutrition

473 calories

- 36g protein
- Carbohydrates - 57g
- Fat - 25g

Prep time + cook time: 20 minutes

Ingredients (for 2 people)

- 100g of quinoa
- 12 deseeded and coarsely chopped red chili
- 1 smashed garlic clove
- 200g of chicken

1 tablespoon extra-virgin olive oil

• 150g roughly sliced tomato

• pitted black kalamata olives, a bunch

• 12 thinly sliced red onion

• 50g crumbled feta cheese

• chopped mint leaves from a small bunch

• 12 lemon juice and zest

Instructions

1. Cook the quinoa according to package directions, then rinse in cool water and completely drain.

2. In the meantime, mix the chicken fillets in olive oil with spice, chili, and garlic. Cook for 3-4 minutes per side in a heated pan, or until cooked through. Place on a platter and put away.

3. Next, combine the tomatoes, olives, onion, feta, and mint in a mixing dish. Add the cooked quinoa. Season thoroughly with the remaining olive oil, lemon

juice, and zest. With the chicken on top, serve.

Day 6: Saturday

Breakfast: Blueberry Oats Bowl

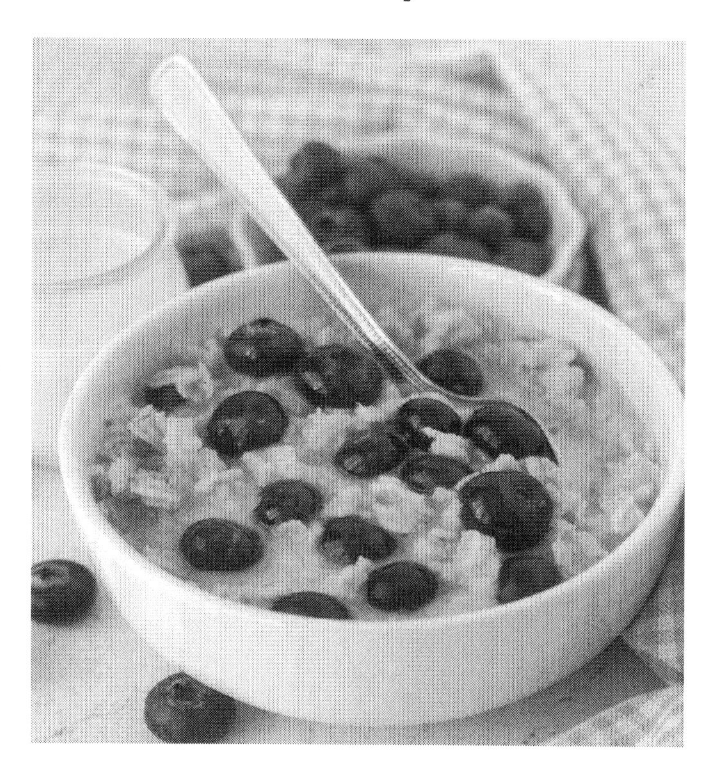

Lunch: Quinoa and Stir Fried Veg

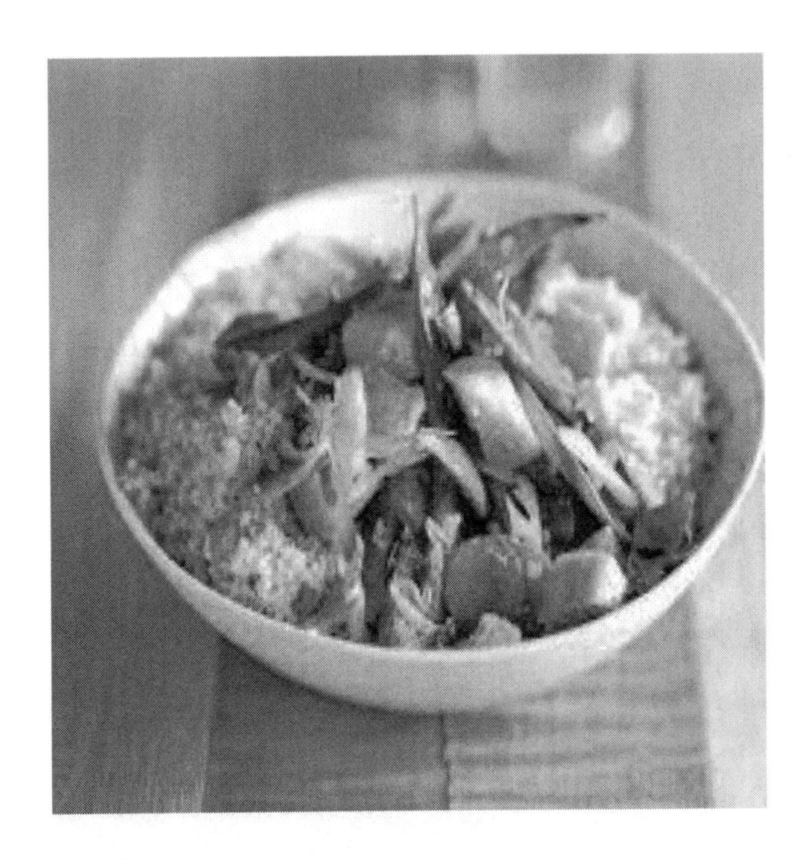

Nutrition

- 473 calories
- 11g protein
- Carbohydrates - 56g
- Fat - 25g

Prep time + cook time: 30 minutes

Ingredients (for 2 people)

- 100g of quinoa
- 3 tablespoons olive oil
- 1 freshly minced garlic clove
- 2 carrot sticks, thinly sliced
- 150g sliced leek

- 150g broccoli, chopped into tiny florets
- 50g tomato
- 100ml vegetable broth
- 1 tablespoon tomato purée
- 1/2 lemon juice

Instructions

1. Prepare the quinoa according per package directions. Meanwhile, in a skillet, heat 3 tbsp of the oil, then add the garlic and briskly sauté for 1 minute. Stir in the carrots, leeks, and broccoli for 2 minutes, or until everything is gleaming.

2. Add the tomatoes, then combine the stock and tomato purée and pour into the pan. Cook for 3 minutes, covered. Toss the quinoa with the remaining oil and lemon juice. Spoon the veggies over top and divide them among heated plates.

Dinner: Grilled Vegetables with Bean Mash

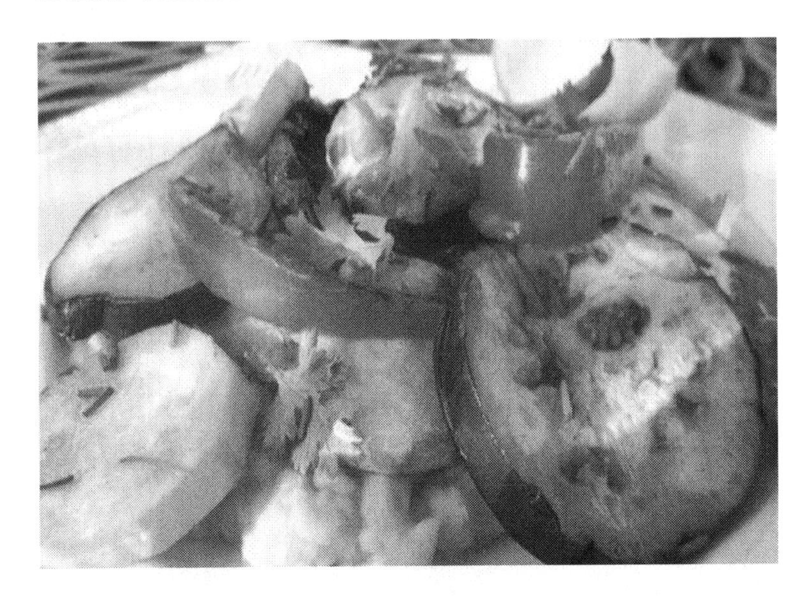

Nutrition

- 314 calories
- 19g protein
- 33g carbs
- Fat - 16g

Prep time + cook time: 40 minutes

Ingredients (for 2 people)

- 1 tablespoon olive oil

- 1 tablespoon red wine vinegar
- 14 teaspoon chili flakes
- 1 tablespoon chopped mint
- 120g chopped tomatoes
- 250g watermelon, diced
- 50g crumbled feta cheese

Instructions

1. Light the grill. Arrange the veggies on a grill pan and gently coat with oil. Cook until lightly browned on one side, then flip and grill until tender on the other.

2. Meanwhile, combine the beans, garlic, and stock in a saucepan. Bring to a boil, then reduce to a low heat and leave uncovered for 10 minutes. Using a potato masher, mash the potatoes coarsely. Divide the mashed veggies across two dishes, drizzle with oil, and season with black pepper and coriander.

Day 7: Sunday

Breakfast: Banana Yogurt Pots

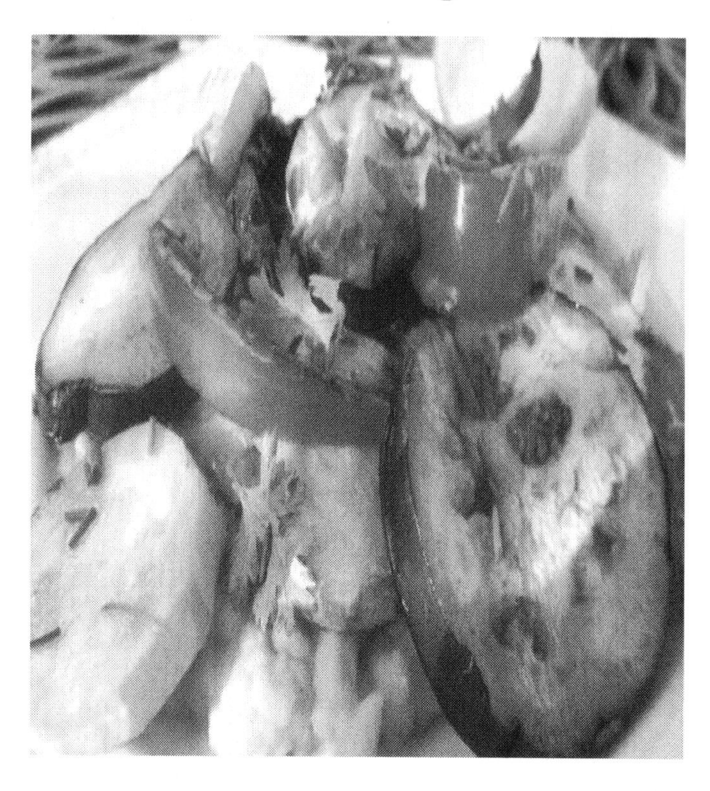

Lunch: Moroccan Chickpea Soup

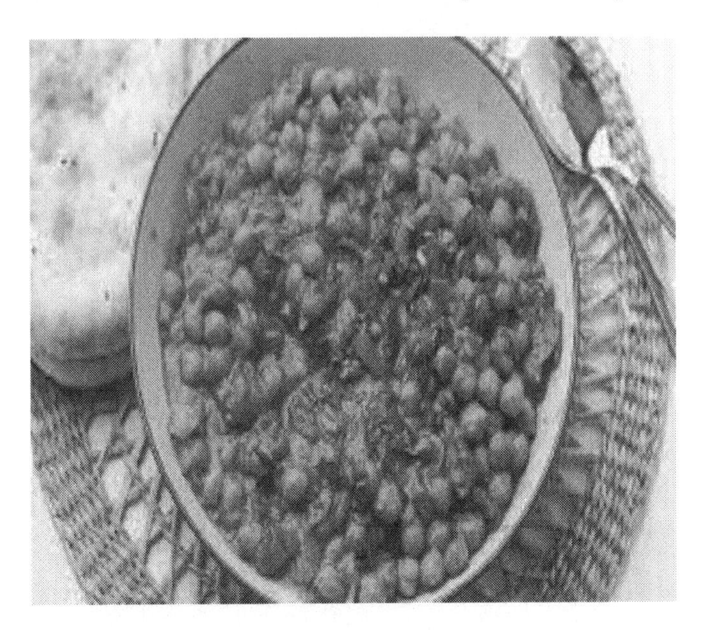

Nutrition

- 408 calories
- 15g protein
- Carbohydrates - 63g
- Fat - 11g

Prep time + cook time: 25 minutes

Ingredients (for 2 people)

- 1 tablespoon olive oil
- 12 medium sliced onion
- 1 sliced celery stick
- 1 teaspoon cumin
- 300ml boiling vegetable stock
- 200g chopped canned tomatoes
- 200g washed and drained chickpeas
- Frozen broad beans (50g)
- 1/2 lemon zest and juice
- coriander and bread for serving

Instructions

1. In a skillet, heat the oil and cook the onion and celery for 10 minutes, or until softened. Fry for another minute after adding the cumin.

2. Increase the heat to high and add the stock, tomatoes, chickpeas, and black pepper. Cook for 8 minutes. Cook for another 2 minutes after adding the wide beans and lemon juice. Serve with lemon zest and coriander on top.

Dinner: Spicy Mediterranean Beet Salad

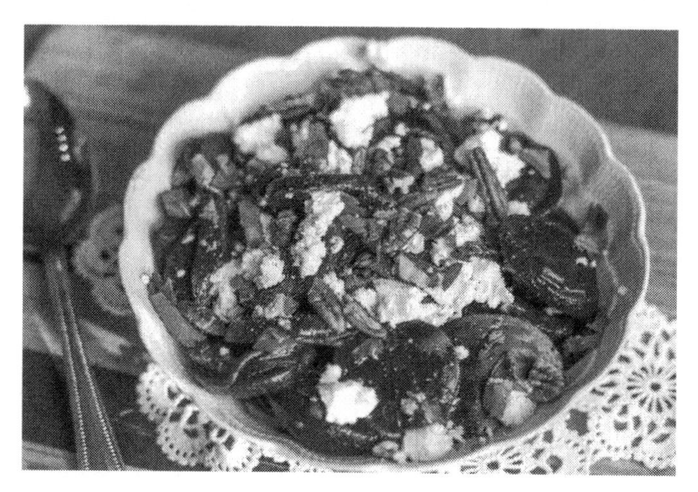

Nutrition

- 548 calories
- 23g protein
- Carbohydrates - 58g
- Fat - 20g

Prep time + cook time: 40 minutes

Ingredients (for 2 people)

- 8 raw baby beetroots or 4 medium cleaned beetroots

- 12 teaspoons za'atar
- 12 tablespoon sumac
- 12 teaspoons of cumin
- 400g drained and washed chickpeas
- 2 tablespoons olive oil
- 12 teaspoons of lemon zest
- 12 teaspoons lemon juice
- 200g plain Greek yogurt
- 1 tablespoon harissa paste
- 1 tablespoon crushed red chili flakes
- chopped mint leaves to serve

Instructions

1. Preheat oven to 220°C/200°C fan/gas mark 1. 7. Depending on size, cut beetroots in half or quarters. Combine the spices. Mix the chickpeas and beets with the oil in a wide baking dish. Season with salt and sprinkle with spices. Mix once more. 30 minutes in the oven

2. Combine the lemon zest and juice with the yogurt while the veggies are cooking. Swirl in the harissa and transfer to a bowl. Sprinkle the chilly flakes and mint over the beets and chickpeas.

Conclusion

If you've had thyroid testing and detected a possible thyroid imbalance, discuss your findings with your healthcare practitioner and find out what next measures they recommend. A balanced diet is a terrific approach to support your general well-being and promote thyroid recovery and wellness. You may be well on your way to a symptom-free lifestyle if you stick to the principles of diet and follow your healthcare provider's particular advice about your individual thyroid issue.

Printed in Great Britain
by Amazon